PROMOTING HAIR GROWTH FOR ALL HAIR TYPES: USING NATURAL METHODS

I0438593

PROMOTING HAIR GROWTH FOR ALL HAIR TYPES: USING NATURAL METHODS

Donna Kakonge

PROMOTING HAIR GROWTH FOR ALL HAIR TYPES: USING NATURAL METHODS

Published by Donna Kay Kakonge, MA, ABD

Toronto, Canada

Library and Archives of Canada

Cataloguing in Publication

Kakonge, Donna Kay Cindy, author

Promoting Hair Growth for All Hair Types: Using Natural Methods

/ Donna Kay Cindy Kakonge.

ISBN 978-1-365-78783-6 | 9781549876387

Copy edit by: Donna Kakonge

Cover illustration by: Donna Kakonge

Printed and Bound in the Canada

SOME BOOKS AND CDS BY DONNA KAKONGE

Headlight Anthology, Vol. 1

What Happened to the Afro?

How to Write Creative Non-fiction

Spiderwoman

My Roxanne

Being Healthy: Selected Works from the Internet (edited by)

Do Not Know

My Story of Transportation

Draft: eSpirituality Chats

Nine (CD)

Journalism Stories Collection

Digital Journals and Numerology

Matoke (Audio Download)

Spiderwoman (Audio Download)

In My Pocket

Where I Was

The Education Generation

Old Romance

How To Start Your Own Teaching and Writing Business

Smoking

The Adventures of a Canvas

Working on My Sleep

Love at a Distance

Teaching Curriculum Ideas

The Politics of Black Hair Online Coursebook

Radio Scripts

Lessons in Public Relations Issues

Totally Unknown Writers Festival Collection 2011 (Published

by Life Rattle Press)

Natural and Colourful Beauty in Education

How To Talk To Crazy People (Published by Life Rattle

Press/Donna Kay Kakonge, M.A. in 2012)

Three Quarters (Donna Kay Kakonge, M.A. in 2014)

Success (Donna Kay Kakonge, M.A. in 2014)

Young Black Women in Toronto High Schools: Portraits of Family, School and Community Involvement in Developing Goals and Aspirations *(Published by Donna Kay Kakonge, M.A. in 2014)*

No Fool No More: Vignettes of Crazy People Talking Sane *(Donna Kay Kakonge, M.A. in 2014)*

Upcoming:

Only My Voice: Vignettes of Crazy People Singing To Stay Sane *(Donna Kay Kakonge, M.A. in 2015)*

God is Always There: Portraits of Family, School and Community Involvement in Developing Goals and Aspirations

Great Fathers, Great Mothers

To the Kakonge Family,

Thank you for showing me so much love.

PREFACE

Hair?

What can it do for you? How does hair make you feel? Do you like your hair? Do you love your hair? Is there something that you want to change about it? Do you like it just the way it is?

This book will give you a perspective on how to improve your hair if this is what YOU desire to do. This book will also help you to grow your hair faster using natural methods if this is what YOU desire to do. This book will also help you to have your hair looking shinier and healthier if this is what YOU desire to do.

If you want all of these thing and for the answers to the above questions to be done in a natural, chemical-free and safe method – read on all my brothers and sisters and transgendered folk from every nationality on earth! I got

something for you!

Über Curly Black Hair

(Don't Worry…read on…the Blondes Are Coming

Too!)

Introduction

I started doing research into the politics of black hair back in 1998. At the time, I was studying at Concordia University in Montréal, Canada doing a master's degree in media studies in the Communications department. This was the beginning of the journey.

While I was in Montréal, I found it difficult to find books that were related to the politics of black hair. I would go to a bookshop in Little Burgundy, a quartier that historically many black people have lived in. A wonderful woman, and I wish I could remember her name, would patiently work with me to order many, many books, mainly from the United States, as well as some from the United Kingdom so I could have material to work with for my research.

My research plan was to do a ninety-page paper, as well as a twenty-six-page website. At the time, I did the website completely by hand, and thanks to that shop in Little Burgundy, my references list for my paper was about five pages long. I graduated in 1999.

Work, writing and teaching eventually led me to start my PhD degree at OISE/University of Toronto in May of 2010 in the Curriculum, Teaching and Learning Development department. The majority of the work that you will see here in this book, including my educational products and acquisitions from taking Foundations of Curriculum with Dr. Heather Sykes, Arts in Education with Dr. Ruben Gaztambide-Fernandez, Introduction to Qualitative Research with Dr. Lance McCready, Black Feminist Thought with Dr. Erica Neegan (who has since changed her last name) and Introduction to Sociological Theory with Dr. Kari Delhi are what you will read here. The inspiration for my forthcoming book with Life Rattle Press that is a creative non-fiction piece dealing with mental health challenges I have had is thanks to my glorious editor Laurie Kallis, and my spectacular professor

of Expressive Writing – Dr. Guy Allen.

The Growth of Black Hair

Black folk, we know, we tend to be particularly susceptible to all of the media hype that surrounds the lies from the haircare industry that a product will make your hair grow. I tell you, I can tell you myself – I have heard it all!

When I was in high school I had a friend of mine who told me that dirt will make your hair grow. Just recently, within the past few years, I had a lover tell me to wash my hair once a month. Yes, he was well-meaning and I listened for a while until my hair felt so bloody nasty that I knew something wrong was going on.

I have had established hairdressers from actually very good salons in the city of Toronto tell me that Coca-Cola has potassium in it and will grow your hair. Fair enough – I do drink Cola because Coca-Cola is too expensive and Cola is basically the same thing so there could be something to that.

I have had wonderful Eritrean, Somali and Ethiopian women tell me that mayonnaise and eggs are good for your hair. This is true my Black folk! It is! I agree. I eat eggs minimum once a week and try to get a little bit of mayonnaise into my diet because I am not as flat stomached as I once was, so I watch it a little bit with the mayo. If you are still young and mainstream beautiful – layer that mayo on my Black friends! Layer it on!

Speaking of which, hair grows its fastest when you are in your twenties. This is a fact. Do take advantage of that.

Another thing for Black folk that also all folk can learn from in fact is how men treat their hair. Men basically do very little with their hair. They cut it; some do not even do that. Women and transgendered people can learn A LOT from men in this regard. Do nothing with your hair, but when it comes to Black hair – condition, condition, condition my friends – natural oils will do that. Do remember to always wash out any conditioner that has instructions that you should wash it out. It can damage your hair if you do not do this. Leave-in conditioners applied first and then applying your hair oil combination should help tremendously, particularly in cold weather seasons or constant cold climates. They also help in warmer climates as well where the heat from the sun will naturally give a hot oil treatment to your hair and your ends and many oils are also good at protecting the colour of your hair against the more fading effects of sunlight.

.

List of Natural Hair Oils Good for Black Folk and Anyone with Naturally Super Curly Hair and What The Oils Do

Note: A good shea butter cream such as Saryna Key if your hair is not in locs/dreads, a good mayonnaise treatment that you can purchase at Loblaws and/or olive oil cream that you can get from Sally's Beauty Supply is a good option to use as a first step after shampooing if your hair is in a natural afro freestyle format.

Almond oil: (basically the same as sweet almond oil), this oil is an essential component to have in your personal apothecary of oils in order to condition your hair.

Amla oil – this oil is what women of Indian descent use on their hair. If you have any Indian in your bloodstream, it is worth it to use this oil.

Argan oil – very good if your hair is a little off-black in colour and/or more brown.

Avocado oil

Bergamot oil – this will cut the scent of oils that a bit more strong in their smell. If you work in such places as a hospital and/or school, you will find this oil complimentary in order to minimize the smells of the combined oils if you choose to use them that way. As well, another tip is that you can apply the oils at night. My sister gave me that very good suggestion.

Castor oil – this is an essential oil! Please listen to what your mothers told you when you were growing up. This oil is good!

Juniper oil – this oil is excellent. It is very conditioning for daily massage oil which you should be doing with your scalp with all of these oils as well as focusing on the ends of your hair.

Lavender oil – not only does this oil have a calm and great scent. It is wonderful for your hair and its balance as well.

Macadamia Nut oil – this is great oil too! Of course, if you are allergic to any nuts and/or nut products, please avoid any oils that contain nuts.

Neem oil – this oil is fantastic! It is Indian oil. It is quite like Buckley's cough syrup in the sense that it smells awful – but, it works! Again if you apply Bergamot oil to a combination of oils that contains neem and apply at night as my sister says it will reduce the scent of the oil.

Olive oil – this is wonderful! I cannot say enough good things about this oil.

Nutmeg oil – again this is good oil, but it contains nuts.

Peppermint oil – this is one of the most important oils you can use! With this oil when you massage it in, you can just feel it stimulate your scalp and promoting hair growth.

Rose/Rosemary oils – not only does this oil smell great, it is good for your hair as well.

Silica oil – this oil is also very, very good, particularly if you have Eastern African heritage.

Tea Tree oil – great for the scalp. Good for massage!

Vanilla oil – this oil is great too!

Walnut oil – another great oil, however again if you are allergic to nuts then you should avoid it.

Note: There are a number of great oils in the Little India Village of Toronto, ON that is also open all-year round that sells a number of great oils that are also complimentary to dark hair types either straight and/or curly.

SHAMPOOING

When should I shampoo my hair? How often should I shampoo my hair? Should I use heat on my hair? Do I need to go to the hairdresser each time I need to get my hair washed?

The answers to these questions are really up to you. I cannot really tell you what to do. A very wise woman who is probably the best loctician in this city, Mariam Ibrahim who also has a book that will give you more knowledge regarding this introductory article, the book being called *Steppin' Out*, told me "just wash your hair when it feels dirty." You see I had asked her all of those above questions and she is right. Everyone does or does not exercise at different levels, everyone does different works and/or works differently even if they are in the same office or wherever is their work location, everyone has different lives to keep all of this simple. It is good to wash your hair everyday if you can. If you have dreadlocks and want your hair to dread quickly, actually the more you wash your hair the faster your hair will dread into mature locs. Also you could try washing your hair every day and if it is not having a damaging effect on your hair but is actually helping your hair, then you know this is the best thing for your hair. Since it seems to make sense for most people, particularly when the weather is hot to wash your skin and your body and brush your teeth every day, it would make sense that as part of your personal hygiene routine that you also wash your hair. The more you get used to it even if you have natural Black hair, you will find it much easier to do. What many people also do and I have also tried this as well is to simply rinse your hair out with water, add condition in order to protect the hair and then go through your usual routine of leave-in conditioner, creams and/or oils if this is part of your grooming ritual. You know your hair best. There is something to be said for hair types. If your hair is drier than it may be a good idea to actually wash your hair with shampoo less. I highly recommend Dr. Bronner's products since these shampoos do not contain foaming agents which will dry out your hair. As well, if your hair is oiler, then you would definitely need to wash your hair more. On the other hand, I have known people with naturally quite oily hair that barely ever wash their hair because they find letting the natural oils nurture their hair is good for their hair and they have long, long beautiful hair to attest to this.

The answer is: "it's up to YOU." Also, the answer is, "wash it when it feels dirty."

What some people do particularly if their hair is very thick is to section the hair with twists and/or braids in order to wash the hair this way. I used to do this in my twenties. Now since my hair is loced I do not really need to do that, however it can be helpful regardless of your hair type.

However, for those who are open to these concepts of the metaphysical sciences, I am about to introduce a concept that is based on numerology that will address your own individual needs in a step-by-step process in order to understand how to deal with your hair at any age:

1. Know your life path number. You can get free information regarding this information at the following website: https://www.decoz.com/. This latter website and numerologist involved Hans Decoz truly is one of the best. He has been studying the art his entire life and he really does know what he is talking about. Born in Holland, there could be some cultural differences in the interpretations, however he is knowledgeable.

2. Once you know your life path number and if you do want to keep your hair for life – this is the following calculation based on time that I would suggest to you that comes from this book: https://www.amazon.ca/dp/B004I6DFSG/ref=dp-kindle-redirect?_encoding=UTF8&btkr=1. It is very good for discussing the timeliness of numerology which is also something good to know that Vedic

Astrologists who mainly come from India know as well.

3. Life path number and hair washing:

-one: wash it yearly for real with soap

-two: you should sprinkle water on your hair to hydrate it on an hourly basis rather engaging in dangerous activities such as smoking cigarettes as just one example – the actual washing should be daily

-three: wash your hair on a monthly basis and/or a little less than a month

-four: you should wash your hair every six months and/or less depending on the above variables that I described above which is in accordance with your lifestyle

-five: you should sprinkle water on your hair on an hourly basis in order to hydrate it and then wash daily

-six: this one is easier to configure – wash on a bi-weekly basis

-seven: wash every week

-eight: is similar to one mentioned above

-nine: wash daily

4. Thank you to Patricia Jarmillo, my neighbor and friend for inspiring this article. I could not have finished this without her.

For more information regarding all of these topics plus a variety of hair types, please check out Mariam Ibrahim's book *Steppin' Out* at: http://www.lulu.com/shop/mariam-ibrahim/stepping-out/paperback/product-18838492.html

YOUR ENDS

Thinking that you need to cut the ends of your hair when they are becoming frazzled is a myth. All you need to do is to apply oils and creams to the end of your hair and condition them well, perhaps a hot oil treatment that focuses on your ends and they will repair.

If you are looking for a good-looking haircut, this is a different story. Yes, of course, you would need to get a good haircut for these purposes. However, if you are looking to grow your hair to lengths which are beyond your dreams – do not, I repeat – do not cut the ends of your hair. Simply condition them as required when you see that your ends need extra care and extra attention. That is all those frazzled ends are telling you.

You have a relationship with your hair. It is on your head every single day. Even for people who are completely bald – that scalp is on your head and wearing you just as much as you are wearing your scalp every day – quotidian as the French would say.

Ensure that because you have a relationship with your hair that you treat the ends of your hair well. You do not need to cut them off as you would cut off a bad friend or bad lover. All you need to do is add extra oil and condition.

This is true of ALL hair types. Even for White folk!

More Exhaustive List of Hair Oils

Here is my list of my personal apothecary of hair oils. Some of them are similar and/or the same as the ones mentioned above. It took me a long time to accumulate this many oils. For you it may take a shorter period of time if this is something that you want. I tend to put all of the oils into my hair and combine them with a clear spray bottle that is rather large from the Dollar Store that I bought for no more than two dollars Canadian. Here is the list. I present this more for me to have a record of what I have than for anything else, as well as knowing that it can also be helpful. I also found Wikipedia to helpful in making up parts of this list or definitely helpful in making in more comprehensive:

Abyssinian oil: also known as crambe seed oil, this oil is considered a new item in the hair oil market. Good for adding moisture and avoiding wrinkles.

Agar oil: also known as oodh and people love how it smells. This one I have yet to own.

Ajwain oil: distilled from leaves. Good for your hair. This one I have yet to own too.

Almond oil: Contains important ingredients such as Omega-3 fatty acids and vitamin E. This oil nourishes and strengthens the hair and is vital for avoidance of hair loss and repairing hair damage.

Aloe Vera oil: helps to treat dry scalp and dandruff for hair. This oil is excellent for growing hair of all hair types. Try to avoid aloe vera gel if you have problems dealing with products that contain alcohol for either your hair and/or skin. The presence of alcohol can have an extremely drying effect on your skin or on your scalp.

Amla oil: this oil is derived from the fruit of an Indian gooseberry. One of the most powerful properties that this particular oil has is that it will darken your hair without the use of hair dyes. This oil would then be ideal for anyone who has naturally dark hair and may be going through that phase of their life when their hair is starting to grey. It also has lots of vitamin C.

Amla Jasmine oil: this oil is very similar to one above, however is specially designed for women who colour their hair.

Angelica Root oil: distilled from a plant. This one I have yet to own too.

Anise oil: used medicinally. Smells like licorice.

Apricot oil: this oil is a good anti-septic and is also an anti-oxidant.

Argan oil: stemming from the Mediterranean, this oil has become increasingly popular among a variety of hair types. It nourishes, adds shines and naturally conditions the hair and the scalp.

Arnica oil: good for the avoidance of acne and chapped skin surfaces. It would help to nourish the scalp for the hair.

Asafoetida oil: used medicinally and to flavor food. Have yet to own.

Avocado oil: has Omega-9 fatty acid and excellent for anti-aging.

Balsam of Peru: from the *Myroxylon*, used in food and drink for flavoring, in perfumes and toiletries for fragrance, and in medicine and pharmaceutical items for healing properties.

Baobob oil: this oil comes from Africa. This oil comes from the Baobob tree. The oil has anti-oxidants, high in vitamin C for skin's elasticity, vitamins A and B for firmer and hydrated skin and Omegas 3, 6 and 9.

Basil oil: this oil is known to be good for reducing anxious feelings and also helpful for diabetes. This is also another essential oil that is good for any oil combination for people from an East Caribbean background.

Bay oil: is used in perfumery; Aromatherapeutic for sprains, colds, flu, insomnia, rheumatism.

Bergamot oil: this oil is great for healing scars that may have been caused to your scalp due to bad chemical treatments; this oil also minimizes the marks on your skin. This oil is also very, very good for reducing the smell of other oils that may have a much stronger and more potent scent.

Birch oil is aromatheapeutic for gout, Rheumatism, Eczema, Ulcers. Do not own.

Black Pepper oil is distilled from the berries of *Piper nigrum.* The warm, soothing effect makes it ideal for treating muscle aches, pains and strains and promoting healthy digestion. Do not own.

Black seed oil: this oil is also known as black cumin, black caraway, black sesame, onion seed and roman coriander. It is seen as curing everything from allergies to hypertension. This is seen as THE best oil in restoring hair loss.

Borage oil: known to be good for inflammation and arthritis, this oil is good for increasing the flexibility of the skin and reducing the pain levels of the skin. This oil would also improve hair growth for a variety of hair types.

Brahmi Amla Herbal Hair oil: coming from a plant that grows in Africa, India and Sri Lanka, this oil can be considered to be a multivitamin for your hair. Good for all hair types.

Calamodin oil or Calamansi Essential Oil comes from a citrus tree in the Philippines extracted via cold press or steam distillation. Do not own.

Calamus oil: used medicinally, in perfumery and (formerly) as a food additive. Do not own.

Camphor oil is used for cold, cough, fever, rheumatism, and arthritis. Do not own.

Cannabis flower essential oil, used as a flavoring in foods, primarily candy and beverages. Also used as a scent in perfumes, cosmetics, soaps, and candles. Do not own.

Canola oil: with Omega fatty acids, this oil can help your hair particularly if your hair is extremely light-coloured.

Caraway oil, used a flavoring in foods. Also used in mouthwashes, toothpastes, etc. as a flavoring agent. Do not own.

Cardamom seed oil, used in aromatherapy and other medicinal applications. Extracted from seeds of subspecies of *Zingiberaceae* (ginger). Also used as a fragrance in soaps, perfumes, etc. Do not own.

Carrot oil: this is great oil for strengthening your hair roots and stimulating hair growth. This is excellent for all hair types.

Castor oil: this oil will promote hair growth and enhance your hair colour. It will also deeply moisturize your scalp.

Cedarwood Virginia oil: there is actually wood in this oil☺. This oil needs to be diluted or it could cause an irritation to your skin.

Chamomile oil: There are many varieties of chamomile but only two are used in aromatherapy; Roman and German. Both have similar medicinal properties but German chamomile contains a higher level of azulin (an anti-inflammatory agent). Do not own.

Chocolate oil: this oil is good for softening the skin on your scalp, as well as literally softening your hair. If you find that you have hard hair that does not tend to be soft, chocolate oil will help to soften it. Combined with vitamin E this oil could be a particularly good alternative for women and men who are in the later part of their lives where the softness of their hair has decreased.

Cinnamon oil: good for stabilizing blood sugar levels and for cardiovascular diseases, this oil has high anti-inflammatory properties. It also helps to heal the skin and/or scalp and works well with carrier oil such as coconut oil.

Cinnamon Bark in Clove oil: Cinnamon Bark oil is good for the immune system. Clove oil eliminates acne, improves blood circulation, reduces gum disease and kills fungus. This is a great oil to have in the oil combination of any hair type.

Citron oil: used in Ayurvedic medicine and perfumery. Do not own.

Citronella oil: from a plant related to lemon grass is used as an insect repellent, as well as medicinally. Do not own.

Clary Sage oil: good for the eyes, nervous system, digestion and kidneys. This helps to promote hair growth for all hair types.

Clove oil: used as a topical anesthetic to relieve dental pain. Do not own.

Coconut oil: helps with the healthy growth of hair and for shinier hair. This oil is also a very good base and/or carrier oil to include with other hair oils that also have a restorative quality to your hair, similar to the effects of olive oil.

Coffee oil: used to flavor food. Do not own.

Coriander oil: Do not own.

Costmary oil (bible leaf oil): formerly used medicinally in Europe; still used as such in southwest Asia. Discovered to contain up to 12.5% of the toxin β-thujone. Do not own.

Costus root oil: used medicinally. Do not own.

Cranberry seed oil: equally high in omega-3 and omega-6 fatty acids, primarily used in the cosmetic industry. Do not own.

Cubeb oil: used medicinally and to flavor foods. Do not own.

Cumin oil/Black seed oil: used as a flavor, particularly in meat products. Also used in veterinary medicine. Do not own.

Curry leaf oil: used medicinally and to flavor food. Do not own.

Cypress oil: used in cosmetics and medicine. Do not own.

Cypriol oil: Do not own.

Davana oil: from the *Artemisia pallens*, used as a perfume ingredient and as a germicide.

Dill oil: chemically almost identical to seed oil.[citation needed] High carvone content. Do not own.

Dudhi Herbal Hair oil: this oil has an extract of dudhi which in Indian Ayurvedic medicine has a natural cooling effect. The oil also has vegetable oil, castor oil and coconut oil in the blend as well.

Elecampane oil: used in herbal medicine. Do not own.

Elemi oil: used as a perfume and fragrance ingredient. Comes from the oleoresins of Canarium luzonicum and Canarium ovatum which are common in the Philippines. Do not own.

Emu oil: Emu oil is particularly good for people with eczema. This oil is good to put in your hair oil combination if you suffer from eczema. It can tend to relieve the condition and/or cure it.

Eucalyptus oil: the eucalyptus tree is an evergreen tree that is native to Australia. This is excellent healing oil. It is good for itchy scalp and gives hair a "pick-me-up." It is also good for all hair types.

Evening Primrose oil: very good for softening the skin. Do not own.

Fennel seed oil: used medicinally, particularly for treating colic in infants. Do not own.

Fenugreek oil: used medicinally and for cosmetics from ancient times. Do not own.

Fir oil: Do not own.

Flaxseed oil: Do not own.

Frankincense oil: this oil comes from the boswellia sacara tree that is normally grown in Somalia. There are also Christian associations with this oil as one of the Wise Men gave

Frankincense to Baby Jesus. It is good for anti-aging and for a scar deterrent.

Galangal oil: used medicinally and to flavor food. Do not own.

Galbanum oil: used in perfumery. Do not own.

Geranium oil: also referred to as Geranol. Used in herbal medicine, particularly in aromatherapy. Also used for hormonal imbalance, for this reason geranium is often considered to be "female" oil. Used in perfumery as well. Do not own.

Ginger oil: this oil is good for pain, an upset stomach, as well as motion sickness. It is also invigorating hair oil that stimulates the scalp in much the same way that peppermint oil does. This is a good hair oil to have for a variety of hair types.

Goldenrod oil used in herbal medicine, including treatment of urological problems. Do not own.

Grapefruit oil, extracted from the peel of the fruit. Used in aromatherapy. Contains 90% limonene. Do not own.

Grapeseed oil: excellent moisturizer for skin and hair.

Guava Seed oil: nourishing and helps to promote hair growth.

Helichrysum oil: Do not own.

Hemani oil: this oil is also known as black cumin, black caraway, black sesame, onion seed and roman coriander. It is seen as curing everything from allergies to hypertension. This is seen as THE best oil in restoring hair loss.

Hempseed oil: good for moisturizing. Do not own.

Henna oil: good for maintaining the colour of your hair.

Hickory nut oil: do not own.

Horseradish oil: do not own.

Hyssop oil: do not own.

Indian Mustard oil: this oil is seen as helpful in stopping grey hair and regrowing hair that is lost.

Jabakusum Herbal Hair oil: a name brand coming from Indian hair oil. Does have coconut oil, olive oil added as well. Advertises that it is meant to add shine and darken dark hair. Some bloggers online are not happy with it, but it does have good ratings on Amazon.com.

Jamaican Rose oil: Rose oil is good as a natural anti-depressant, however for your hair it is a very good anti-bacterial medicinal element to include in your hair oil combination.

Jasmine oil: used for its flowery fragrance.

Jojoba oil: Jojoba oil is great for smoothing the frizz from curly hair and just as overall great conditioning oil. It also works well as a base and/or carrier oil to support other oils that also have positive effects towards hair.

Juniper oil: Juniper oil from the Juniper berry can calm and ground and has a more aromatherapy effect to hair than a more growing effect on hair. It is good to add to a hair combination as well. I have also read that this particular oil is good to put into the oil combinations of people with Eastern Caribbean backgrounds.

Kukui Nut oil: this oil is from an official tree in Hawaii. This is excellent for dry hair and dry scalp.

Lavender oil: this is the most used oil in the world. Its anti-oxidant properties are wonderful for hair and skin.

Lemon oil: nourishes the skin and the hair.

Lemongrass: Lemongrass is a highly fragrant grass from India. In India, it is used to help treat fevers and infections. The oil is very useful for insect repellent. Do not own.

Lime oil: this oil has a lot of vitamin C in it. You can avoid dandruff and bring life to dull, frizzy or oily hair with lime oil.

Liquid Lanolin oil: this is sheep sebum. On the technical side, it is considered to be a wax. When it comes in oil form, it can have the same nourishing effect on or with your hair as castor oil.

Linaloe: do not own.

Macadamia Nut oil: this oil is good for sensitive skin, good for mature skin and has a calming effect. Good for all hair types.

Mahabhringraj Tail oil: this oil promotes hair growth and hair strength. If you already have grey hair, this oil is very, very good for helping your existing grey hair to look very healthy.

Mandarin: do not own.

Marjoram: a very good oil. This one I have too.

Marula oil: a good oil for when you are on holiday to help with the sunshine and its effect on colouring your hair. Also good for helping with chlorinated pools and sea salts from the swimming in the sea.

Mehndi oil: the same as henna oil.

Melaleuca: same as Tea Tree oil.

Melissa oil (Lemon balm): sweet smelling oil used primarily medicinally, particularly in aromatherapy. Do not own.

Mentha arvensis oil: Mint oil, used in flavoring toothpastes, mouthwashes and pharmaceuticals, as well as in aromatherapy and other medicinal applications.

Mineral oil: this oil stems from petroleum. For the hair it is used as a moisturizer and a lubricant.

Moringa oil: this oil comes from the moringa oleifera tree. Makes for a suppler scalp and stronger hair, fights dandruff and split ends.

Mountain Savory: do not own.

Mugwort oil: used in ancient times for medicinal and magical purposes. Currently considered to be a neurotoxin. Do not own.

Mustard oil: this oil is seen as helpful in stopping grey hair and regrowing hair that is lost. The only difference between this oil and the Indian mustard oil is that this particular oil is not particularly for people of Indian descent or have Indian heritage.

Myrrh oil: warm, slightly musty smell. Used medicinally.

Myrtle oil: do not own.

Navratna oil: prevents hair loss, good for avoiding dandruff and promoting hair growth.

Neem oil: not only is neem oil so potent that is effective in killing pests, but is also extremely good for the health of your hair. It does everything that every other oil says it does – this is excellent hair oil. It does have a very, very strong odour. The use of bergamot mentioned earlier with this oil would be a good idea if you work in a setting where odour is an issue.

Neroli oil: this oil relieves heart palpitations and has calmed, relaxing effect. This oil has also been known to be good in relieving the effects of menopause. It also repairs and rejuvenates skin and works similar to orange oil and it is for this latter reason why it is good for any hair oil combination.

Nutmeg oil: coming from Indonesia, Malaysia and Sri Lanka, this oil is good for massaging your scalp in order to promote hair growth.

Olive oil: this oil comes from a traditional tree crop in the Mediterranean. This is very good carrier oil for your hair that can be used in conjunction with other oils.

Oil of Oregano oil: this oil has anti-oxidant properties and can be good for the hair as well.

Oontanga oil: this oil comes from the Kalahari Desert and has a beautiful scent as many of the oils do. It is very good for balancing the natural oils of your hair.

Orange oil: known to have cancer-fighting properties that also boost the immune system, this oil is good to have in your hair oil combination.

Orris oil: is extracted from the roots of the Florentine iris (*Iris florentina*), *Iris germanica* and *Iris pallida*. It is used as a flavouring agent, in perfume, and medicinally. Do not own.

Palo Santo: I own this oil. It is good for the hair.

Parsley oil: used in soaps, detergents, colognes, cosmetics and perfumes, especially men's fragrances. Do not own.

Patchouli oil: natural anti-septic that is therapeutic to have in an oil combination with coconut, olive oil, jojoba oil as carrier oils.

Peanut oil: very rich in vitamin E, it is very, very important that any products that contain nuts, including any aforementioned products that contain nuts are not used by yourself if you have allergies to nut products.

Peppermint oil: many people discuss how powerful mint and peppermint can be as a healing power. This oil is great for stimulating the scalp and for scalp massages. You can feel your scalp tingle as soon as you apply this oil. Great for keeping away mice too.

Perilla essential oil: extracted from the leaves of the perilla plant. Contains about 50–60% perillaldehyde. Do not own.

Petitgrain: do not own.

Pimento oil: anti-septic and anti-oxidant effect, this is a good oil to have as part of your oil combination.

Pine oil: used as a disinfectant, and in aromatherapy. Do not own.

Pomegranate Seed oil: very nourishing and healthy attributes to contribute to your hair.

Ravensara: a very good oil.

Red Cedar: do not own.

Roman Chamomile: do not own.

Roop oil: good for prevention of acne, also good to have in a hair combination.

Rose oil: distilled from rose petals, Used primarily as a fragrance.

Rosehip oil: distilled from the seeds of the *Rosa rubiginosa* or *Rosa mosqueta*. Used medicinally.

Rosemary oil: balances the hormonal levels within the body, this oil are good as an anti-inflammatory as well. It is good to have as a part of your hair oil combination and for other health properties as many of the oils in this list.

Rosemary French oil: this oil stimulates cell growth and reduces the lines of mature skin. This oil is good for a variety of hair types in their hair oil combination.

Rosewood oil: used primarily for skin care applications. Also used medicinally.

Sage oil: used medicinally.

Sandalwood oil: used primarily as a fragrance, for its pleasant, woody fragrance.

Safflower oil: very good for people particularly of East African descent, or with very dark and very curly hair.

Sapote oil: this oil comes from Mexico and Central America and good for both dry and oily hair. Contains vitamins A, B, C, D and E.

Sassafras oil: from sassafras root bark. Used in aromatherapy, soap-making, perfumes, and the like. Formerly used as a spice, and as the primary flavoring of root beer, *inter alia*. Sassafras oil is heavily regulated in the United States due to its high safrole content. Do not own.

Savory oil: from *Satureja* species. Used in aromatherapy, cosmetic and soap-making applications. Do not own.

Schisandra oil: used medicinally.

Sesame oil: eliminates hair loss and is good for stimulating hair growth.

Shea Butter oil: this is a lot of vitamin A and vitamin E in shea butter oil. The oil is wonderful to put in hair and is extremely nourishing for naturally curly hair types of all different hair colours.

Shikaka Herbal Hair oil: this is Indian oil that contains a lot of the aforementioned Indian oils.

Silica oil: not a lot is written online about this oil. The one that I have is derived from a flower and also bach flowers. It smells wonderful and seems to have nothing to do with silicone oil, although the names are similar. This oil is wonderful and very nourishing for the hair. It also smells great.

Spearmint oil: often used in flavoring mouthwash and chewing gum, among other applications. Do not own.

Spikenard oil: used medicinally. Do not own.

Spruce oil: has calming and elevating properties. It can be used as a topical application for muscular aches and pains, poor circulation, and rheumatism. Spruce Oil has also been used to improve breathing conditions of asthma, bronchitis, coughs, and general weakness. Do not own.

Star anise oil: highly fragrant oil using in cooking. Also used in perfumery and soaps, has been used in toothpastes, mouthwashes, and skin creams. Ninety percent of the world's star anise crop is used in the manufacture of Tamiflu, a drug used to treat influenza, and is hoped to be useful for avian flu.

Sweet Almond oil: rich in vitamin E, this oil is wonderful for nourishing all hair types and is a wonderful oil to have in your hair oil combination.

Sunflower oil: with Omegas 9 and 6, plus loaded with vitamin E, this oil is particularly good for people with lighter hair shades.

Tangerine oil: do not own.

Tarragon oil, distilled from *Artemisia dracunculus*, used medicinally. Do not own.

Tamanu oil: the tamanu tree resides in Southeast Asia. This does contain nut products.

Tea Tree Oil: this oil is good for everything from insect bites to psoriasis. Used as a natural astringent for your scalp, this is a very good hair oil to have in the oil combination of any skin type.

Thyme oil: this oil kills infections and helps to balance the hormonal levels of an individual. This oil is good for all hair types.

Tsuga oil: belongs to the pine tree family. It is used as analgesic, antirheumatic, blood cleanser, and stimulant. It treats cough, respiratory conditions, kidney ailments, urinary infections. Do not own.

Turmeric oil: used medicinally and to flavor food. Do not own.

Valerian oil: is used for insomnia, migraines, nervous dyspepsia. Do not own.

Vanilla oil: has nourishing qualities to all hair types.

Vetiver oil: (khus oil) a thick, amber oil, primarily from India. Used as a fixative in perfumery, and in aromatherapy.

Vitamin A oil: vitamin A is great for anti-aging. The oil also works well with the health of your hair.

Vitamin D3 oil: this is good for adding lustre and health to your hair. It is also good for managing the effects that sunlight has on your tresses.

Vitamin E oil: containing natural anti-oxidants, vitamin E oil is also great anti-aging oil. This is a particularly good oil to have in your hair oil combination if you are starting to see grey hairs in your head☺.

Walnut oil: great oil for hair.

Warionia: used as a perfume ingredient among local women. Do not own.

Western red cedar: do not own.

Wheat Germ oil: this oil has the highest concentration of vitamin E outside vitamin E oil itself. This oil is particularly good for those people with lighter shaded hair.

Wintergreen oil: can be used as an analgesic, anodyne, anti rheumatic & anti arthritic, anti spasmodic, anti septic, aromatic, astringent, carminative, diuretic, emenagogue and stimulant. Do not own.

Yarrow oil: is used medicinally to relieve joint pain. Do not own.

Ylang Ylang oil: this essence is commonly used in many shampoos and is known for promoting the health of hair.

Zedoary oil: used medicinally and to flavor food. Do not own.

Footnote: If you live in a cold climate and your oils happen to get congealed because of the cold in your living situation, if you have a microwave about twenty seconds inside there should be enough to bring the oil(s) back to its liquid form. If you do not own a microwave and I know some people do not like them, you can just let the oil sit on your countertop for no longer than one day and by this time the oil will liquefy. You may need a spend a tad bit more on the heat and turn up the heat in your home to speed this up if you keep your place particularly cold.

USING HEAT

I understand that some people just must use heat. After washing their hair, their hair needs to be dry fast and I understand that the fastest way to dry your hair is to use heat.

What I do is to let my hair air dry. I really find this to be the best thing to do.

Heat can be really, really damaging to every single type of hair. I do understand that if you just absolutely need to use your hair dryer – then, yes, please do continue to use it.

I have found that it is best that if you can resist heat, do so. Heat does come in handy if you have a heating cap and you can add a combination of the oils mentioned above for your hair type and go for a hot oil treatment with the heating cap in order to nourish your hair further. So, I am not completely against heat.

What to Do With These Oils for Maximum Effect?

The best way to use the oils for maximum effect is to combine all of the oils that you know will have the best effect for your hair. There are also many other oils that I have not mentioned so you may want to do more research about this and as I come up with more oils I will also add to the list.

For financial reasons and since oils can be expensive you may only want to invest in the cost of the oils that are the best for your hair type. You should purchase a clear or opaque spray bottle from a store such as the Dollar Store and add the oils about half way in the bottle. Fill the rest of the bottle with water. Each time that you use the oil and water combination, make sure that you shake the bottle so that the oil and water are well combined.

Oil and water do mix. You just need to shake the combination of the oil and the water and then it will mix. This will add the best effect for your hair with the oils and the water and keep your hair very healthy. Do not forget to also massage your scalp daily to promote hair growth.

SWIMMING

Swimming is a great form of exercise, however unless you are swimming in a fresh water lake and/or the sea, if you are swimming in a chlorinated pool – you need to protect your hair or the chlorine will ruin it.

Neutrogena puts out a great Anti-Residue shampoo that will help to completely cleanse your hair after you have gone swimming. Prior to swimming, I would recommend that you use a very heavy leave-in conditioner of your choice in order to protect your hair and please do not forget to wash your hair as soon as you can in a comfortable environment after you have finished the joy of swimming. It is a wonderful activity to be involved in and just some precautions to keep your hair looking good will ensure that you do not need to stop this enjoyable activity because of what it is doing to your skin and hair.

A quick mention as well to ensure your skin does not start to flake from the effects of chlorine – ensure that you lubricate your skin with a choice skin cream after you have completed each session of your swimming. Chlorine can also be very tough on your skin, and also on your nails. It is not the water that is a problem – it is the chlorine. However, chlorine is necessary and mandatory to have for the public health element of public swimming pools.

Wearing Protective Styles

Most women and men are the Kings and Queens on how to wear protective styles in between washing, or when hair is wet, or when you are trying to set a style or you just want to do something different, or you are protecting your hair while doing any form of exercise.

There is not much I can add to your own inner intuition. Let it Flow!

Hats and Wraps

Sometimes a great-looking hat or even a toque can get you looking and feeling just great. Make sure that you are careful about how much you wear them. It is true that wearing a hat too much and too often can restrict the blood vessels in your scalp and inhibit the growth of your hair. There are certain days, of course when it is not extremely cold outside when you can forgo wearing a hat or wrap.

If this is your religion – personally I support that. Ignorant governments have no right based on any universal law to tell someone else how to dress as long as they are dressed!

.

Note About Locs and Dreads

What does fall down, can be re-attached my loced brothers and sisters. Since hair does shed, it is only normal that your locs could break off – I would suggest that you simply re-attach it. I just tie it on right back into my hair since I do not really tend to tie anything else on since I have not had an alcoholic drink since 2004.

The other option is to sew the loc(s) back into your hair – which is absolutely fine. Of course you would want to use a thread that is similar to your natural hair colour unless you are trying to make a fashion statement – understood and supported on my part.

Bear in mind that even when you look on Google Images, the majority of first images that you see of dreadlocks are of White people with dreadlocks and I think they look equally as beautiful as the dreadlocks on Black people. Just like when a Black person, usually the women, has a straight relaxer style that looks really good and she has paid the money to have it done well – her hair can look just as good as any White folk out there.

All of you of any racial persuasion – continue to go on with your bad selves!

Colouring Your Hair – Safe Ways to Colour Hair

In general, my rule of thumb is not to colour your hair if you can. Colouring your hair can have many, many damaging effects on your hair that are extremely visible until new growth of a good length appears that has not been coloured.

I know for everyone this is not an option, however I really do think that if you know the colouring of your hair is damaging your hair then you should stop the colouring of your hair. Henna has been known to do wonderful things and a woman once told me that she went to Ethiopia it was just a marvel to see all the beautiful Ethiopian women with Henna in their hair with the kind of pure light that the country receives. I do understand why a lot of people want to colour their hair.

There is also this woman who I did a story on while I was a journalist at the CBC who was an expert colourist. She worked at Civello Salon and used Aveda products which singer Lauryn Hill helped to make famous. This expert colourist really did a fabulous job on colouring the hair of many different people. It is worth it if you can afford it to spend the money for an expert colourist to colour your hair. This way you will also ensure that it not only looks good, but is also healthy for your hair.

Locing and/or Dreading Your Hair

So many people have great stories to tell about their hair locing journey. Although I had a fantastic hair loctician Mariam Ibrahim help me start my locs and she had encouraged me to do so for four years before I made the final decision to loc, I will always be grateful for her time, her kindness and her tremendous skills.

If you live in a part of the world where it could be difficult for you to find a loctician, one way you can start your locs would be to do it on your own.

You do not need nor require beeswax, however if this is your choice to use this – it will help your hair to loc faster and that is true! I used beeswax to loc my hair in the late nineteen nineties and my hair loced instantaneously! Although beeswax can sometimes dull the look of your natural hair so you must keep re-applying. It is generally recommended for those people who have a Caucasian hair type that they do use beeswax to loc their hair because it is more difficult and takes longer in order to loc that hair type.

If you have hair that is more African such as mine, then you could either put your hair in two strand twists, or even three linked braids and just let nature do its thing. Be mindful of the hair washing schedule mentioned above and you should be able to see beautiful results in a matter of six months guaranteed after you start your locs. Once locs reach about the one or two year mark, they are in their teenage years and once they are three to four years old, they are more mature locks.

Some ways of maintaining your mature locks rather than getting sick of them and just cutting them off would be to choose some styles such as updos, etc. and visit a good loctician in order to get your hair styled so that you can have your hair off your face and do something different with your hair. This will help to not ever have an end for how long you will wear your locs.

Going Natural

Fallacy number one: you can go natural even though you have straightened or relaxed hair at your ends. Meaning you can do this! You would just need to be really, really delicate with the point where your natural hair ends and your relaxed hair ends off your hair. Very delicate!

My hair has been completely natural – no relaxer since nineteen-ninety-three. A few things I have learned is that the advice in the Lonnice Brittenum Bonner series of books if followed, does work. During my twenties my hair was down into my back and I broke bad habits by spending time having my hands in my hair and twisting and untwisting and then retwisting again to get that neo-dread look so that my hair could look like that beautiful singer Des'ree whose music I did and still do love so much.

Then, I went to a salon in Montréal and I know the people were actually well-meaning, however they told me that

I should use conditioner and not wash it out. They did not know any better. I did not know any better. My back-length neo-dreads broke off to a more Grace Jones inspired look.

Telling you that if you want long hair – do not do this! The only conditioners that you should leave into your hair are those which specifically indicate that it is a leave-in conditioner.

Natural hair is very easy to maintain. If you use a good leave-in conditioner that will accentuate your curls, plus oils if you choose to, and also wash your hair when it is best for you – it will grow and you will see wonderful results with your natural hair.

Preserving Your Natural Hair Colour of all Hair Types

Not only is this wonder vitamin good for preserving your natural hair colour, it is also good for your nails, teeth and skin. What is it?

It's vitamin E.

Whether you take it as a liquid, whether you use it topically as an oil or take capsules of vitamin E or even make that added effort to eat and drink those grocery store products that contain a lot of vitamin E – you will be doing yourself good. This goes for both women and men.

Vitamin E can help to slow down the growth of grey hair, or also help to make your existing grey hair look healthier.

Vitamin E can help your skin look younger and healthier, plus your nails and teeth too. Fluoride that you get at the dentist and in toothpaste has a lot of vitamin E.

Deciding to Shave it All Off – What is it with this Bothersome Nuisance called Hair? ☺

Nothing is wrong in deciding to keep your hair either very, very low or even shaving it off completely. Many people do not even have a choice in this matter, so it can be completely understood. There are many famous female singers who have even made shaved heads sleek, cool and dare I say sexy. Here are some of them to name a few:

- Meshell Ndegeocello

- Grace Jones

- Sinead O'Connor

All extremely beautiful women who sometimes even looked better off without hair than with. If you know that you have a face of an angel and you really just do not want to bother with the sometimes nuisance of hair – go for it! I support you!

Keeping Your Scalp Nice and Clean and Looking Attractive

Keeping your shaven scalp looking nice and clean and attractive involves washing your scalp based on the schedule previously mentioned, plus applying a good leave-in conditioner that you should massage into your scalp daily. Trust me – I do know. My head has been bald once too ☺. I could not even believe that one of my prettiest friends at the time said "you look good." I still cannot figure out if she was telling the truth or we were really that good friends!

Good Times to Cut your Hair and/or Your Nails –
Towards Growth (if this is what you prefer because there
really is something that you need to cut out of your life ☺
LOL)

As mentioned on the numerological scale above, I will
now let you know the timing that is involved based on the day
that you choose to go for a haircut (if you really feel that you
need one and natural oils will not help your ends):

One Days: If you have super curly hair and you get a
major cut of hair on your own personal number one day, do
not expect your hair to fully show any significant growth for
about a year or less. However, if you do not really want to see
your hair grow that fast because as an example and of course
using a stereotype (sorry) you are a man in a job where a short
haircut is necessary for your image – choosing personal one
days would work to your advantage because then you would
not need to go to the barber often at all.

Two Days: If it is a two day, your hair will start slowly growing literally within an hour after the haircut. This is a good day if you want to see rapid length repair after the haircut.

Three Days: About a month later you will start to see the hair growth.

Four Days: This will take about six months or less.

Five Days: Works like the two days – you will see growth very soon.

Six Days: This is good too. About two weeks later you will see growth to your hair.

Seven Days: This is good too and a number that many people like. About a week later this is when you will start to see growth to the hair.

Eight Days: Works like the one; you will not see any significant growth until about a year later.

Nine Days: It works like the three – it will take about a month.

Being an Overnight Guest and How to Take Care of

Your Skin, Nails and Hair

So I will simply address this question not based on all
the various scenarios that could be linked to this one, but
focus on three scenarios: you are sleeping over at a platonic
friend's place, you are sleeping over at a family's house, you
are sleeping over at a non-platonic friend's place. Let's start
with the first one.

You are young, still under forty years of age and still too
young to be sleeping over at a non-platonic friend's place.
What do you do? It's a sleep-over and how you going to show
off your beauty when the sun rises in the morning?

First of all, if you are allowed to because water is
expensive for most people – use their shower. Do not use
soap. Wash your self gently with the water and you could also
cleanse your hair, but just do nothing to it until you get home
so that you can use your own products. What I do is keep

some oils on me so I can use that as a leave-in conditioner. If you have a favourite one and the bottle is too big to drag around, try to put a little bit in a bag even and do not forget to follow the original instructions and then wash it out.

For family, as a general rule and if you choose to, you can then use what your family has to cleanse yourself. You are all in the same bloodline – at least most of it. If you are not – nurture has made you like blood any way.

A non-platonic friend works the same way as a friend – well, not really, but I hope you understand the context I mean within the focus of this book.

Pets and Hair

I had this beautiful cat that was in a traumatic situation before I received him. On one side of his neck the fur was all scratched off from his own nails because the people who had him before would leave him alone for days on end and then the alarm bells would go off in the previous owner's apartment building and this would just drive the cat Lance crazy.

When I first got Lance, he would hide from me. I could spend close to thirty minutes searching for him throughout my apartment and then end up finding him under my bed hiding from me. The kind veterinarian not too far from where I live told me that Lance needed to re-establish his sense of trust, as well as needed good cat food to help his fur to grow back.

At the point I had Lance it was the early millennium and I paid almost twenty dollars a bag for the cat food! This is how much I loved Lance! However, the kind veterinarian knew what she was talking about – Lance's fur grew back and he stopped his habit of clawing at his neck and started coming up to me to cuddle.

I share this experience with you because if there is an animal in your life who you love and you want to ensure that their fur and also their overall health is just superb – please visit your local veterinarian. We have a lot of great ones out there!

References

Abreu, J. (2009). On Kids Transformed by Music. TED Talks. [Video].

Addams, J. (1908). The public school and the immigrant child. Ch 3 in Flinders, David & Thornton, Stephen. (Eds.) The curriculum studies reader, 2nd ed New York: Routledge.

http://simplelink.library.utoronto.ca/url.cfm/84091

Aker, J.C. and I.M. Mbiti. (March/April 2010). "Africa Calling: Can Mobile Phones Make a Miracle?" Boston Review. [Internet].

http://bostonreview.net/BR35.2/aker_mbiti.php

Amoah, J. (2007). "Building Sandcastles in the snow; Meanings and Misconceptions of the development of Black Feminist Theory in Canada," in *Theorizing Empowerment:*

Canadian Perspectives on Black Feminist Thought, pp. 95-118 2. Inanna Publications, Toronto.

Arie.I. (January, 1990). "I Am Not My Hair," *Testimony Vol.1*, 2006. Album.

Butt, Richard, Townsend, David and Danielle Raymond. "Bringing Reform to Life: teacher's stories and professional development," *Cambridge Journal of Education.* Routledge: January, 1990.

Baker, B. (2002). The hunt for disability: The new eugenics and the normalization of school children. Teachers College Record, 104(4), 663-703.

http://simplelink.library.utoronto.ca/url.cfm/83929

Benjamin, W. (1968). The work of art in the age of mechanical reproduction. In

Illuminations, (pp. 217-251). New York: Schocken Books [Available Online]

Bobbit, F. (1918). Ch VI Scientific method in curriculum-making. In The Curriculum (pp. 41-52). Boston, MA: Houghton Mifflin.

http://simplelink.library.utoronto.ca/url.cfm/60614

[also printed in: Bobbit, Franklin. (1918/2004). Scientific method in curriculum-making. Ch 1 in Flinders, David & Thornton, Stephen. (Eds.) The curriculum studies reader, 2nd ed New York: Routledge.

http://simplelink.library.utoronto.ca/url.cfm/84091

Bogdan, R. & Biklen, S. (2003). "Developing Analytic Questions" and "Examples of Observational Questions for Educational Settings," in

Qualitative research for education: An introduction to theories and methods. Toronto: Pearson Education Group.

Braverman. H. (1998) *Labor and Monopoly Capital: The degradation of Work in the Twentieth Century* (25th Anniversary Edition) New York: Monthly Review Press. (chapters 1-4; chapter 20 is supplemental) [pdf provided]

Britzman, D. (1998). Queer pedagogy and its strange techniques. Ch 4 in Lost subjects, contested objects (pp. 79-95). New York: SUNY.

http://simplelink.library.utoronto.ca/url.cfm/85865

❦ Britzman, D. Early days of critical pedagogy in relation to psychoanalysis. Video on The Paulo and Nita Friere International Project for Critical Pedagogy.

http://www.freireproject.org/content/critical-pedagogy-tv

Broido, E. and Manning, K. (2002). Philosophical Foundations and Current Theoretical Perspectives in Qualitative Research. Journal of College Student Development, 43 (4), 434-445.

Buckingham, D. (2003). Media education and the end of the critical consumer.

Harvard Educational Review, 73(3), 309-327.CIA.gov. (N/A). "The World Factbook – Telephones – Mobile Cellulair." [Internet].

https://www.cia.gov/library/publications/the-worldfactbook/rankorder/2151rank.html

Butt, R., Townsend, D. and Raymond, D. (1990). Bringing reform to life: Teachers' stories and professional development. Cambridge Journal of Education, 20(3), 225-268.

http://simplelaink.library.utoronto.ca/url.cfm/83909

Butterfield, J. (2010). From the Soul COLOURblind 2010 Royal Ontario Museum. [Art Exhibit].

Carr, W. & Kemmis, S. (1986/2002). Teachers, Researchers and Curriculum. Ch 1 in Becoming critical: Education, knowledge and action research. New York: Routledge/Falmer.

[Available as e-Book in UofT library]

http://simplelink.library.utoronto.ca/url.cfm/83908

CBC.ca. (2010). "Contact Us." [Internet].

http://www.cbc.ca/contact/

Cole, P. & O'Riley, P. (2002). Much rezadiuex about (Dewey's) goats in the curriculum. Ch 4 in Doll, William & Gogh, Noel. Curriculum Visions (pp. 123-150). New York: Peter Lang.

http://simplelink.library.utoronto.ca/url.cfm/83912

Connell, R. (2009). Gender research: Five examples. In Gender: Short introductions (13-30). Cambridge, UK: Polity Press.

Collins, P. H. (March 2000). "Gender Black Feminism, and Black Political Economy." The Annals of the American Academy of Political and Social Science 568 (March 2000): 41-53. Reprinted in The Study of African American Problems: W.E.B. Du Bois's Agenda, Then and Now, eds. Elijah Anderson, and Tukufu Zuberi, (Thousand Oaks, CA: Sage, Publications).

Craig, M.L. (2002). Ain't I a Beauty Queen?: Black Women, Beauty and the Politics of Race. USA: Oxford University Press.

Craig, M. L. (1997). "The Decline and the Fall of the Conk; or, How to Read a Process," in Fashion Theory: The Journal of Dress, Body and Culture vol 1. Issue 4. New York: Berg Publishers.

Creswell, J. W. (2007). Qualitative inquiry & research design: Choosing among the five approaches (2nd ed.). Thousand Oaks, CA: Sage.

Davies, B. (2003). Ch 1 Poststructuralist theory and the study of gendered childhoods. Shards of glass: Children reading and writing beyond gendered identities. Cresskill, NJ: Hampton.

Davies, B. (2003). Ch 8 Writing beyond the male-female binary. Shards of glass: Children reading and writing beyond gendered identities. Cresskill, NJ: Hampton.

Dewey, J. (1934/2005). *Art as Experience.* New York: Perigee [AE].

Dewey, J. (1929/2004). My pedagogic creed. The curriculum studies reader, 2nd ed (pp. 17-24). New York: Routledge.

http://simplelink.library.utoronto.ca/url.cfm/84091

DuBois, W.E.B. (1903/1990). The Training of the Black man. Ch 6 in The Souls of Black Folk. (pp. 62-76) New York: Vintage.

http://simplelink.library.utoronto.ca/url.cfm/84837

Ellis, G. (2010). Till I'm Laid to Rest. Nsemia Press, Oakville, Canada.

Ellsworth, E. (1989). Why doesn't this feel empowering? Working through the repressive myths of critical pedagogy. Harvard Educational Review, 59(3), 297-324.

http://simplelink.library.utoronto.ca/url.cfm/85834

Friere, P. (1970). Pedagogy of the oppressed. Ch 12 in Flinders, David & Thornton, Stephen. (Eds.) The curriculum studies reader, 2nd ed New York: Routledge.

http://simplelink.library.utoronto.ca/url.cfm/84091

http://simplelink.library.utoronto.ca/url.cfm/27659

Gray, M. Singer/Actress.

Gutierrez, K. (2009). Looking for educational equality: Immigrants, migrants and the new Latino diaspora. School of Education Videos, Syracuse University.

http://soeweb.syr.edu/video/index.cfm?videoID=7

Henry, A. (1998). Taking Back Control: African Canadian women teachers' lives and practice. Albany: State University of New York.

hooks, b. (2002). Be Boy Buzz. Illus. C. Raschka. New York: Hyperion. (from Wheeler and Sword).

hooks, b. (2000). Art is for everybody. In D. Chasman and E. Chian (eds.), Drawing us in, (pp. 96-104). Boston: Beacon.

hooks, b. (2000). *Art is for everybody.* In D. Chasman and E. Chian (eds.), *Drawing us in*, (pp. 96-104). Boston: Beacon.

hooks, b. (1999). Happy to be Nappy. New York: Hyperion Books for Children.

hooks, b. (1994). Outlaw culture: Resisting representation. London: Routledge.

hooks, b. (1994). Eros, eroticism and the pedagogical process. Ch 13 in Teaching to Transgress (pp. 191-199).

hooks, b.   (1995). "Black Beauty and Black Power: Internalized Racism." Killing Rage: Ending Racism.   New York: Henry Holt and Company.

hooks, b. (1994). Theory as liberatory practice. Ch5 in Teaching to transgress: Education as the practice of freedom. (pp. 59-76). New York: Routledge.

hooks, b.   (1993).   Sisters of the Yam: black women and self-recovery. Toronto: Between the Lines.

hooks, b. (1992). Black Looks : Race and Representation. Toronto : Between the Lines.

hooks, b. (1990). Yearning : Race, Gender, and Cultural Politics. Boston : South End Press.

hooks, b. (1989). Talking back: Thinking feminist, thinking black. Boston: South End.

hooks, b. (1988). "Straightening Our Hair." Z Magazine (Sept.):33-37.

Kakonge, D. (2010). "Black Woman with Afro embodied by a Rose and Based in Water," *Donna Magazine*. [Internet – October 27, 2010].

http://kakonged.wordpress.com/2010/10/21/painting-of-black-woman-with-afro-embodied-by-a-rose-and-based-in-water-is-art/

Kakonge, D. (2008). "Matoke," *Spiderwoman*. 3rd ed. Self-Published, 2008.

Kakonge, D. (2007). *Spiderwoman*. Lulu.com: Self-Published.

Kakonge, D. (2002). "John Ware, February 2002 for CBC Syndication National Radio News," Donna Magazine. [Internet].
http://kakonged.wordpress.com/2009/05/08/josiah-henson-%E2%80%93-february-2002-for-cbc-syndication-national-radio-news/

Kakonge, D. (2000). "What Happened to the Afro?" Donna Magazine. [Internet].
http://kakonged.wordpress.com/2008/02/16/68/

Kakonge, D. (1995). "Listen 'in (Defunct Proposal to the CBC) – Selections from Upcoming Book Stories in Red and Yellow," Donna Magazine. [Internet].

http://kakonged.wordpress.com/2009/07/25/listenin-defunct-proposal-to-the-cbc/

Kanu, Y. & Glor, M. (2006). 'Currere' to the rescue? Teachers as 'amateur intellectuals; in a knowledge society. Journal of the Canadian Association for Curriculum Studies, 4(2), 101-122.

http://simplelink.library.utoronto.ca/url.cfm/83911

🎥Kincheloe, J. Interviewed. Video on The Paulo and Nita Friere International Project for Critical Pedagogy.

http://www.freireproject.org/content/joe-kincheloe-interviewed

Kincheloe, J. (2008). Ch 1 Introduction (pp. 1-43). Critical pedagogy primer. New York: Peter Lang.

Kincheloe, J. (2008). Ch 2 Foundations of critical pedagogy (pp. 45-96). Critical pedagogy primer. New York: Peter Lang.

Kleibard, H. (1975). The rise of scientific curriculum making and its aftermath. Curriculum Theory Network, 5(1), 27-38.

http://simplelink.library.utoronto.ca/url.cfm/83882

Lashua, B. (2006). "Just another Native'? Soundscapes, Chorasters, and Borderlands in Edmonton, Alberta, Canada. Cultural Studies – Critical Methodologies, 6(3), 391-410

Lemert C. (2002). "Poetry and Public Life." *Cultural Studies/Critical Methodologies,* Volume 2 Number 3: 371-393.

Lensmire, T. (2008). How I became White while punching de Tar Baby. *Curriculum Inquiry*, 38(3), 299-322.

Leonardo, Z. (2002). The Souls of White Folk: Critical pedagogy, whiteness studies and globalization discourse. Race, ethnicity and education. 5(1), 29-50.
http://simplelink.library.utoronto.ca/url.cfm/84836

Lloyd, J. (October 23, 2010). [Phone Message-Transcription].

Micallef, S. (2003). Murmur Project. [Internet].
http://murmurtoronto.ca/

Lorde, A. (1968/1984). Poetry is Not a Luxury. In *Sister Outsider: Essays and Speeches*, (pg. 36-39). New York: Norton, Quality Paperback Book Club.

Marson, U. (1931). *Kinky Hair Blues*. Kingston: Gleaner.

Massaquoi, N. and Wane, N. (2007). Theorizing Empowerment: Canadian Perspectives on Black Feminist Thought. Inanna Publications: Toronto.

McCready, L. (2004). Some challenges facing queer youth in urban high schools: Racial segregation and de-normalizing whiteness. Journal of Gay and Lesbian Issues in Education, 1(3), 37-51.

http://simplelink.library.utoronto.ca/url.cfm/85868

McIntosh, P. (1988). "White Privilege and Male Privilege: A Personal Account of Coming to See Correspondences Through Work in Women's Studies." *Working Paper No. 189*. Wellesley Center for Research on Women.

Memmi A. (1957/1969). *The Colonizer and the Colonized*. Introduction by Jean-Paul Sartre. Boston: Beacon Press. (several copies in U of T libraries, as well as google books).

Miller, S. and Parker, B.A. (2009). "Reframing the Power of Lesbian Daughters' Relationships With Mothers Through Black Feminist Thought." Journal of gay & lesbian social services 21.2: 206-218.

Mills, C. W. (1959). "The Promise." In *The Sociological Imagination* (pp. 3-24). New York: Oxford University Press.

Morrow, W. (1973). *400 Years Without a Comb*. San Diego, California: Black Publishers.

Newton-John, O. (2004). "Let's Get Physical," Physical, 1981. Album.

Pinar, William. "Autobiography: A revolutionary act. Ch 2" What is curriculum theory? (pp. 35-62). Mahwah, NJ: Lawrence Erlbaum Press.

Oregon Public Broadcasting. (1997). *A World of Art: Works in Progress.* Annenberg Media Initiative. Mierle Ukeles.

Oshibanjo, R. (2006). Do You Hair Me? The Politics of Black Hair Online Course. July 19, 2010 to present. http://affiliate.kickapps.com/_Do-You-Hair-Me/blog/2631461/107952.html

Phoenix, A. (2004). Neoliberalism and masculinity: Racialization and the contradictions of schooling for 11 to 14 year olds. Youth and Society, 36(2), 227-246.

http://simplelink.library.utoronto.ca.myaccess.library.utor
onto.ca/url.cfm/85538

Pinar, W. (2004). Autobiography: A revolutionary act. Ch
2 in What is curriculum theory? (pp. 35-62). Mahwah, NJ:
Lawrence Erlbaum Press.

Pinar, W. (1975). The method of "Currere". Paper
presented to the American Research Association, Washington,
DC. April. ERIC document 104 766.

Popkewitz, T. (2004). The alchemy of mathematics
curriculum: Inscriptions and the fabrication of the child.
American Educational Research Journal, 41(1), 3-34.
http://simplelink.library.utoronto.ca/url.cfm/83926

Rattan, J. (October 23, 2010). [Phone Message-
Transcription].

Razack, S. (2005). "How White Supremacy is Embodied: Sexualized Racial Violence at Abu Ghraib." *Canadian Journal of Women and the Law* 17 (2): 341-363.

Razack, S. (1998). Looking White People in the Eye: Gender, Race and Culture in Courtrooms and Classrooms. Toronto: University of Toronto.

Rock, C. (2009). Good Hair. [Documentary].

Rogers, J. (1985). *The Dictionary of Clichés*. New York: Ballantine Books.

Rooks, N. M. (2004). Ladies' Pages: African American Women's Magazines and the culture that made them. London: Rutgers Press.

Rooks, N. M. (1996). Hair raising : beauty, culture, and African American women. New Jersey : Rutgers University Press.

Quigley, D. (N/A). "Dealing with Technology in the Classroom," Teachervision. [Internet].
http://www.teachervision.fen.com/internet-safety/teacher-tips/63634.html

Richardson, V. (2003). Constructivist pedagogy. Teachers College Record, 105(9), 1623-1640.
http://simplelink.library.utoronto.ca/url.cfm/83927

Russell, K,, Wilson, M., and Hall, R. (1992). *The Color Complex*. New York, Anchor.

Scott, J. Singer/Actress.

Schwab, J. (1969). The practical: A language for curriculum. School Review, 78(1), 1-23.

http://simplelink.library.utoronto.ca/url.cfm/83858

Simpson, D. (2001). John Dewey's Concept of the Student. Canadian Journal of Education, 26(2), 183-200.

http://simplelink.library.utoronto.ca/url.cfm/83884

Soul II Soul. (1989). "Keep on Moving," Club Classics Vol. One. UK: London.

Special Issue on Critical Pedagogy. Educational Theory, (1998), 48(4), 431-462. [Available online at Uof T library]

http://simplelink.library.utoronto.ca/url.cfm/84046

Theme Issue: Rethinking Social Reproduction. Interchange, (1981), 12(2-3). (For articles by Henry Giroux, Micheal Apple and Paul Willis.)

http://simplelink.library.utoronto.ca/url.cfm/84045

Springgay, S. (2008). Body knowledge and curriculum: Pedagogies of touch in youth and visual culture. NY: Peter Lang.

Tate, S. A. (2009). Black Beauty: Aesthtics, Stylization, Politics. London: Ashgate Publishing Ltd.

Tate, S. A. (2005). Black Skins, Black Masks: Hybridity, Dialogism, Hybridity. London: Ashgate Publishing Ltd.

Tate, S. A. (2000). "Looking for identity: Is it possible to find 'hybridity' in Black people's narratives?" in Roots and Rituals: the construction of ethnic identities, eds. Dekker, T. J.

The Artist Formerly Known as Prince. (1984). "The Beautiful Ones," *Purple Rain*. Los Angeles, USA: Warner Bros.

The Canadian Press. (September 15, 2010). "Schools should be Open to Cellphones in Class," Toronto: Globe and Mail. [Internet].

http://www.theglobeandmail.com/news/national/ontario/schools-should-be-open-to-cellphones-in-class-mcguinty/article1708313/

Titchkosky T. & Michalko R. (2009), "Introduction" to *Rethinking Normalcy: A Disability Studies Reader*, Edited by Tanya Titchkosky and Rod Michalko. Toronto: Canadian Scholars Press.

Tyler, R. (1957). The curriculum – Then and now. The Elementary School Journal, 57(7), 364-374.

http://simplelink.library.utoronto.ca/url.cfm/83853

Wallace, M. (1990). *Invisibility Blues*. Edmonton: Alpine Press Inc.

Weiler, K. (2001). Rereading Paulo Friere. In Weiler, Kathleen. (Ed.), Feminist engagements: Reading, resisting and revisioning male theorists in education and cultural studies. http://simplelink.library.utoronto.ca/url.cfm/57214

Williams and Chau (2007). "Notes on Feminism, Racism and Sisterhood," in *Theorizing Empowerment: Canadian Perspectives on Black Feminist Thought* pp. 285-295. Inanna Publications, Toronto.

Willis, P. (1990). Symbolic creativity. In Common culture: Symbolic work at play in the everyday cultures of the young, (pp. 1-29). Buckingham, UK: Open University Press.

Fieldnotes

Lethal Beauty – Global Friday, September 10, 2010 – Skin Deep Database

Ariel Fenster-McGill – Cosmetics

CTV – James contacted you @ SSHRC – story on evening news @ cosmetics danger

Glamour Gals – Salon 4 tweens

8.5 billion in sales tweens – by 2012

Skincare education by the age of 5

ACKNOWLEDGEMENTS

Thank you to Dr. Sam Kakonge, Dr. Guy Allen, Dr. David Goldberg, Dr. Kwai Li, Dr. Antoinette Gagné, Dr. Njoki Wane, Dr. Ann Lopez, Dr. Laura Lush, Dr. Merlin Charles, Teresa Madaleno-Long, Kitty Salsberg, Marion Gold and my readers and encouraging friends and family and nieces. I also thank myself. We should all thank ourselves, especially when we are doing productive things that help us to live healthy, sane and life-affirming lives. I am still learning though, I am still learning.

www.ingramcontent.com/pod-product-compliance
Lightning Source LLC
Chambersburg PA
CBHW020519290526
45786CB00002B/680